Date: ....

Quote Of The Day

Today I am truly grateful for...

Here's what would make today great...

I am...

Some amazing things that happened today...

Some amazing things that happened today...

What could I have done to make today even better?

Date: ______________

Quote Of The Day

Today I am truly grateful for...

Here's what would make today great...

I am...

Some amazing things that happened today...

Some amazing things that happened today...

What could I have done to make today even better?

Date: _______________________

Quote Of The Day

Today I am truly grateful for...

Here's what would make today great...

I am...

Some amazing things that happened today...

Some amazing things that happened today...

What could I have done to make today even better?

Date:

Quote Of The Day

Today I am truly grateful for...

Here's what would make today great...

I am...

Some amazing things that happened today...

Some amazing things that happened today...

What could I have done to make today even better?

Date:

Quote Of The Day

Today I am truly grateful for...

Here's what would make today great...

I am...

Some amazing things that happened today...

Some amazing things that happened today...

What could I have done to make today even better?

Date:

Quote Of The Day

Today I am truly grateful for...

Here's what would make today great...

I am...

Some amazing things that happened today...

Some amazing things that happened today...

What could I have done to make today even better?

Date: _______________

Quote Of The Day

____
____

Today I am truly grateful for...

____
____
____
____

Here's what would make today great...

____
____
____
____

I am...

____
____

Some amazing things that happened today...

____
____

Some amazing things that happened today...

____
____

What could I have done to make today even better?

____

Date: _______________

Quote Of The Day

____
____

Today I am truly grateful for...

____
____
____
____
____

Here's what would make today great...

____
____
____
____
____

I am...

____
____
____

Some amazing things that happened today...

____
____

Some amazing things that happened today...

____
____

What could I have done to make today even better?

____
____

Date:

Quote Of The Day

Today I am truly grateful for...

Here's what would make today great...

I am...

Some amazing things that happened today...

Some amazing things that happened today...

What could I have done to make today even better?

Date: ....

Quote Of The Day

Today I am truly grateful for...

Here's what would make today great...

I am...

Some amazing things that happened today...

Some amazing things that happened today...

What could I have done to make today even better?

Date:

Quote Of The Day

Today I am truly grateful for...

Here's what would make today great...

I am...

Some amazing things that happened today...

Some amazing things that happened today...

What could I have done to make today even better?

Date: _______________

Quote Of The Day

Today I am truly grateful for...

Here's what would make today great...

I am...

Some amazing things that happened today...

Some amazing things that happened today...

What could I have done to make today even better?

Date:

Quote Of The Day

Today I am truly grateful for...

Here's what would make today great...

I am...

Some amazing things that happened today...

Some amazing things that happened today...

What could I have done to make today even better?

Date: ______________________

Quote Of The Day
____
____
____

Today I am truly grateful for...
____
____
____
____
____

Here's what would make today great...
____
____
____
____
____

I am...
____
____
____

Some amazing things that happened today...
____
____

Some amazing things that happened today...
____
____
____

What could I have done to make today even better?
____
____

Date:

Quote Of The Day

Today I am truly grateful for...

Here's what would make today great...

I am...

Some amazing things that happened today...

Some amazing things that happened today...

What could I have done to make today even better?

Date:

Quote Of The Day

Today I am truly grateful for...

Here's what would make today great...

I am...

Some amazing things that happened today...

Some amazing things that happened today...

What could I have done to make today even better?

Date: _______________

Quote Of The Day

Today I am truly grateful for...

Here's what would make today great...

I am...

Some amazing things that happened today...

Some amazing things that happened today...

What could I have done to make today even better?

Date: ....

Quote Of The Day

Today I am truly grateful for...

Here's what would make today great...

I am...

Some amazing things that happened today...

Some amazing things that happened today...

What could I have done to make today even better?

Date: ____________________

Quote Of The Day

Today I am truly grateful for...

Here's what would make today great...

I am...

Some amazing things that happened today...

Some amazing things that happened today...

What could I have done to make today even better?

Date: _______________

Quote Of The Day

Today I am truly grateful for...

Here's what would make today great...

I am...

Some amazing things that happened today...

Some amazing things that happened today...

What could I have done to make today even better?

Date: ____________________

Quote Of The Day

____
____
____

Today I am truly grateful for...

____
____
____
____
____

Here's what would make today great...

____
____
____
____
____

I am...

____
____

Some amazing things that happened today...

____
____

Some amazing things that happened today...

____
____

What could I have done to make today even better?

____
____

Date: _______________

Quote Of The Day

Today I am truly grateful for...

Here's what would make today great...

I am...

Some amazing things that happened today...

Some amazing things that happened today...

What could I have done to make today even better?

Date:

Quote Of The Day

Today I am truly grateful for...

Here's what would make today great...

I am...

Some amazing things that happened today...

Some amazing things that happened today...

What could I have done to make today even better?

Date: ....

Quote Of The Day

____
____
____

Today I am truly grateful for...

____
____
____
____
____

Here's what would make today great...

____
____
____
____
____
____
____

I am...

____
____
____

Some amazing things that happened today...

____
____

Some amazing things that happened today...

____
____

What could I have done to make today even better?

____
____

Date:

Quote Of The Day

Today I am truly grateful for...

Here's what would make today great...

I am...

Some amazing things that happened today...

Some amazing things that happened today...

What could I have done to make today even better?

Date:

Quote Of The Day

Today I am truly grateful for...

Here's what would make today great...

I am...

Some amazing things that happened today...

Some amazing things that happened today...

What could I have done to make today even better?

Date: _______________

Quote Of The Day
____
____
____

Today I am truly grateful for...
____
____
____
____
____

Here's what would make today great...
____
____
____
____
____

I am...
____
____
____

Some amazing things that happened today...
____
____

Some amazing things that happened today...
____
____

What could I have done to make today even better?
____
____

Date: ______________

Quote Of The Day

____
____

Today I am truly grateful for...

____
____
____
____

Here's what would make today great...

____
____
____
____

I am...

____
____

Some amazing things that happened today...

____

Some amazing things that happened today...

____
____

What could I have done to make today even better?

____
____

Date:

Quote Of The Day

Today I am truly grateful for...

Here's what would make today great...

I am...

Some amazing things that happened today...

Some amazing things that happened today...

What could I have done to make today even better?

Date: ....

Quote Of The Day

Today I am truly grateful for...

Here's what would make today great...

I am...

Some amazing things that happened today...

Some amazing things that happened today...

What could I have done to make today even better?

Date: _______________

Quote Of The Day

____

____

____

Today I am truly grateful for...

____

____

____

____

____

Here's what would make today great...

____

____

____

____

____

I am...

____

____

Some amazing things that happened today...

____

____

Some amazing things that happened today...

____

____

What could I have done to make today even better?

____

Date: ....

Quote Of The Day

Today I am truly grateful for...

Here's what would make today great...

I am...

Some amazing things that happened today...

Some amazing things that happened today...

What could I have done to make today even better?

Date: ....

Quote Of The Day

Today I am truly grateful for...

Here's what would make today great...

I am...

Some amazing things that happened today...

Some amazing things that happened today...

What could I have done to make today even better?

Date: ....

Quote Of The Day

Today I am truly grateful for...

Here's what would make today great...

I am...

Some amazing things that happened today...

Some amazing things that happened today...

What could I have done to make today even better?

Date: _______________

Quote Of The Day

____
____

Today I am truly grateful for...

____
____
____
____
____

Here's what would make today great...

____
____
____
____
____

I am...

____
____

Some amazing things that happened today...

____
____

Some amazing things that happened today...

____
____

What could I have done to make today even better?

____

Date: _______________________

Quote Of The Day

Today I am truly grateful for...

Here's what would make today great...

I am...

Some amazing things that happened today...

Some amazing things that happened today...

What could I have done to make today even better?

Date: ....

Quote Of The Day

Today I am truly grateful for...

Here's what would make today great...

I am...

Some amazing things that happened today...

Some amazing things that happened today...

What could I have done to make today even better?

Date:

Quote Of The Day

Today I am truly grateful for...

Here's what would make today great...

I am...

Some amazing things that happened today...

Some amazing things that happened today...

What could I have done to make today even better?

Date:

Quote Of The Day

Today I am truly grateful for...

Here's what would make today great...

I am...

Some amazing things that happened today...

Some amazing things that happened today...

What could I have done to make today even better?

Date:

Quote Of The Day

Today I am truly grateful for...

Here's what would make today great...

I am...

Some amazing things that happened today...

Some amazing things that happened today...

What could I have done to make today even better?

Date: _______________

Quote Of The Day

____

____

____

Today I am truly grateful for...

____

____

____

____

____

Here's what would make today great...

____

____

____

____

____

I am...

____

____

Some amazing things that happened today...

____

____

Some amazing things that happened today...

____

____

What could I have done to make today even better?

____

____

Date: ....

Quote Of The Day

____
____
____

Today I am truly grateful for...

____
____
____
____
____

Here's what would make today great...

____
____
____
____
____

I am...

____
____
____

Some amazing things that happened today...

____
____

Some amazing things that happened today...

____
____

What could I have done to make today even better?

____
____

Date:

Quote Of The Day

Today I am truly grateful for...

Here's what would make today great...

I am...

Some amazing things that happened today...

Some amazing things that happened today...

What could I have done to make today even better?

Date: ....

Quote Of The Day

____

____

Today I am truly grateful for...

____

____

____

____

Here's what would make today great...

____

____

____

____

I am...

____

____

____

Some amazing things that happened today...

____

____

Some amazing things that happened today...

____

____

What could I have done to make today even better?

____

____

Date: _______________

Quote Of The Day

____
____
____

Today I am truly grateful for...

____
____
____
____
____

Here's what would make today great...

____
____
____
____
____

I am...

____
____
____

Some amazing things that happened today...

____
____

Some amazing things that happened today...

____
____
____

What could I have done to make today even better?

____
____

Date: ....

Quote Of The Day

Today I am truly grateful for...

Here's what would make today great...

I am...

Some amazing things that happened today...

Some amazing things that happened today...

What could I have done to make today even better?

Date:

Quote Of The Day

____

Today I am truly grateful for...

____

Here's what would make today great...

____

I am...

____

Some amazing things that happened today...

____

Some amazing things that happened today...

____

What could I have done to make today even better?

____

Date: ....

Quote Of The Day

Today I am truly grateful for...

Here's what would make today great...

I am...

Some amazing things that happened today...

Some amazing things that happened today...

What could I have done to make today even better?

Date:

Quote Of The Day

Today I am truly grateful for...

Here's what would make today great...

I am...

Some amazing things that happened today...

Some amazing things that happened today...

What could I have done to make today even better?

Date: ___________________

Quote Of The Day

____
____
____

Today I am truly grateful for...

____
____
____
____
____

Here's what would make today great...

____
____
____
____
____
____

I am...

____
____
____

Some amazing things that happened today...

____
____

Some amazing things that happened today...

____
____

What could I have done to make today even better?

____
____

Date:

Quote Of The Day

Today I am truly grateful for...

Here's what would make today great...

I am...

Some amazing things that happened today...

Some amazing things that happened today...

What could I have done to make today even better?

Date: ....

Quote Of The Day

Today I am truly grateful for...

Here's what would make today great...

I am...

Some amazing things that happened today...

Some amazing things that happened today...

What could I have done to make today even better?

Date: _______________

Quote Of The Day

Today I am truly grateful for...

Here's what would make today great...

I am...

Some amazing things that happened today...

Some amazing things that happened today...

What could I have done to make today even better?

Date:

Quote Of The Day

Today I am truly grateful for...

Here's what would make today great...

I am...

Some amazing things that happened today...

Some amazing things that happened today...

What could I have done to make today even better?

Date:

Quote Of The Day

Today I am truly grateful for...

Here's what would make today great...

I am...

Some amazing things that happened today...

Some amazing things that happened today...

What could I have done to make today even better?

Date: ....

Quote Of The Day

Today I am truly grateful for...

Here's what would make today great...

I am...

Some amazing things that happened today...

Some amazing things that happened today...

What could I have done to make today even better?

Date: ....

Quote Of The Day

____
____
____

Today I am truly grateful for...

____
____
____
____
____

Here's what would make today great...

____
____
____
____
____

I am...

____
____
____

Some amazing things that happened today...

____
____

Some amazing things that happened today...

____
____

What could I have done to make today even better?

____
____

Date: ....

Quote Of The Day

Today I am truly grateful for...

Here's what would make today great...

I am...

Some amazing things that happened today...

Some amazing things that happened today...

What could I have done to make today even better?

Date: _______________

Quote Of The Day

Today I am truly grateful for...

Here's what would make today great...

I am...

Some amazing things that happened today...

Some amazing things that happened today...

What could I have done to make today even better?

Date: _______________

Quote Of The Day

____

____

Today I am truly grateful for...

____

____

____

____

Here's what would make today great...

____

____

____

____

I am...

____

____

Some amazing things that happened today...

____

____

Some amazing things that happened today...

____

____

What could I have done to make today even better?

____

____

Date: ______________________

Quote Of The Day

____

____

Today I am truly grateful for...

____

____

____

____

Here's what would make today great...

____

____

____

____

____

I am...

____

____

Some amazing things that happened today...

____

Some amazing things that happened today...

____

____

What could I have done to make today even better?

____

____

Date: ....

Quote Of The Day

Today I am truly grateful for...

Here's what would make today great...

I am...

Some amazing things that happened today...

Some amazing things that happened today...

What could I have done to make today even better?

Date: ....

Quote Of The Day

Today I am truly grateful for...

Here's what would make today great...

I am...

Some amazing things that happened today...

Some amazing things that happened today...

What could I have done to make today even better?

Date:

Quote Of The Day

____

Today I am truly grateful for...

____

Here's what would make today great...

____

I am...

____

Some amazing things that happened today...

____

Some amazing things that happened today...

____

What could I have done to make today even better?

____

Date: _______________

Quote Of The Day
____
____

Today I am truly grateful for...
____
____
____
____

Here's what would make today great...
____
____
____
____

I am...
____
____

Some amazing things that happened today...
____
____

Some amazing things that happened today...
____
____

What could I have done to make today even better?
____
____

Date: ....

Quote Of The Day

Today I am truly grateful for...

Here's what would make today great...

I am...

Some amazing things that happened today...

Some amazing things that happened today...

What could I have done to make today even better?

Date:

Quote Of The Day

Today I am truly grateful for...

Here's what would make today great...

I am...

Some amazing things that happened today...

Some amazing things that happened today...

What could I have done to make today even better?

Date: ....

Quote Of The Day

Today I am truly grateful for...

Here's what would make today great...

I am...

Some amazing things that happened today...

Some amazing things that happened today...

What could I have done to make today even better?

Date: ....

Quote Of The Day

Today I am truly grateful for...

Here's what would make today great...

I am...

Some amazing things that happened today...

Some amazing things that happened today...

What could I have done to make today even better?

Date: ___________________________

Quote Of The Day
____
____
____

Today I am truly grateful for...
____
____
____
____
____

Here's what would make today great...
____
____
____
____
____

I am...
____
____
____

Some amazing things that happened today...
____
____

Some amazing things that happened today...
____
____

What could I have done to make today even better?
____
____

Date: _______________

Quote Of The Day
____
____

Today I am truly grateful for...
____
____
____
____

Here's what would make today great...
____
____
____
____

I am...
____
____

Some amazing things that happened today...
____
____

Some amazing things that happened today...
____
____

What could I have done to make today even better?
____
____

Date: _______________

Quote Of The Day

____
____
____

Today I am truly grateful for...

____
____
____
____
____

Here's what would make today great...

____
____
____
____
____
____

I am...

____
____
____

Some amazing things that happened today...

____
____

Some amazing things that happened today...

____
____

What could I have done to make today even better?

____
____

Date:

Quote Of The Day

Today I am truly grateful for...

Here's what would make today great...

I am...

Some amazing things that happened today...

Some amazing things that happened today...

What could I have done to make today even better?

Date: ....

Quote Of The Day

Today I am truly grateful for...

Here's what would make today great...

I am...

Some amazing things that happened today...

Some amazing things that happened today...

What could I have done to make today even better?

Date: _______________

Quote Of The Day

____
____

Today I am truly grateful for...

____
____
____
____

Here's what would make today great...

____
____
____
____

I am...

____
____

Some amazing things that happened today...

____
____

Some amazing things that happened today...

____
____

What could I have done to make today even better?

____

Date: ....

Quote Of The Day

____

____

Today I am truly grateful for...

____

____

____

____

Here's what would make today great...

____

____

____

____

I am...

____

____

Some amazing things that happened today...

____

____

Some amazing things that happened today...

____

____

What could I have done to make today even better?

____

____

Date: ....

Quote Of The Day

Today I am truly grateful for...

Here's what would make today great...

I am...

Some amazing things that happened today...

Some amazing things that happened today...

What could I have done to make today even better?

Date: _______________

Quote Of The Day

____
____
____

Today I am truly grateful for...

____
____
____
____
____

Here's what would make today great...

____
____
____
____
____
____

I am...

____
____
____

Some amazing things that happened today...

____
____

Some amazing things that happened today...

____
____

What could I have done to make today even better?

____
____

Date:

Quote Of The Day

Today I am truly grateful for...

Here's what would make today great...

I am...

Some amazing things that happened today...

Some amazing things that happened today...

What could I have done to make today even better?

Date: _______________

Quote Of The Day

____
____
____

Today I am truly grateful for...

____
____
____
____
____
____

Here's what would make today great...

____
____
____
____
____
____
____

I am...

____
____
____

Some amazing things that happened today...

____
____

Some amazing things that happened today...

____
____

What could I have done to make today even better?

____
____

Date:

Quote Of The Day

Today I am truly grateful for...

Here's what would make today great...

I am...

Some amazing things that happened today...

Some amazing things that happened today...

What could I have done to make today even better?

Date: ....

Quote Of The Day

Today I am truly grateful for...

Here's what would make today great...

I am...

Some amazing things that happened today...

Some amazing things that happened today...

What could I have done to make today even better?

Date: ....

Quote Of The Day
____
____
____

Today I am truly grateful for...
____
____
____
____
____

Here's what would make today great...
____
____
____
____
____

I am...
____
____
____

Some amazing things that happened today...
____
____

Some amazing things that happened today...
____
____
____

What could I have done to make today even better?
____
____

Date: _______________

Quote Of The Day

____
____

Today I am truly grateful for...

____
____
____
____

Here's what would make today great...

____
____
____
____
____

I am...

____
____
____

Some amazing things that happened today...

____
____

Some amazing things that happened today...

____
____

What could I have done to make today even better?

____
____

Date: ....

Quote Of The Day

____
____
____

Today I am truly grateful for...

____
____
____
____
____

Here's what would make today great...

____
____
____
____
____
____

I am...

____
____
____

Some amazing things that happened today...

____
____

Some amazing things that happened today...

____
____

What could I have done to make today even better?

____
____

Date: ____________

Quote Of The Day

Today I am truly grateful for...

Here's what would make today great...

I am...

Some amazing things that happened today...

Some amazing things that happened today...

What could I have done to make today even better?

Date:

Quote Of The Day

Today I am truly grateful for...

Here's what would make today great...

I am...

Some amazing things that happened today...

Some amazing things that happened today...

What could I have done to make today even better?

Date: _______________________

Quote Of The Day

____
____
____

Today I am truly grateful for...

____
____
____
____
____
____

Here's what would make today great...

____
____
____
____
____
____
____

I am...

____
____
____

Some amazing things that happened today...

____
____
____

Some amazing things that happened today...

____
____
____

What could I have done to make today even better?

____
____

Date:

Quote Of The Day

Today I am truly grateful for...

Here's what would make today great...

I am...

Some amazing things that happened today...

Some amazing things that happened today...

What could I have done to make today even better?

Date: ______________________

Quote Of The Day

Today I am truly grateful for...

Here's what would make today great...

I am...

Some amazing things that happened today...

Some amazing things that happened today...

What could I have done to make today even better?

Date: ....

Quote Of The Day

____

____

Today I am truly grateful for...

____

____

____

____

Here's what would make today great...

____

____

____

____

I am...

____

____

Some amazing things that happened today...

____

____

Some amazing things that happened today...

____

____

What could I have done to make today even better?

____

____

Date:

Quote Of The Day

Today I am truly grateful for...

Here's what would make today great...

I am...

Some amazing things that happened today...

Some amazing things that happened today...

What could I have done to make today even better?

Date: ....

Quote Of The Day

Today I am truly grateful for...

Here's what would make today great...

I am...

Some amazing things that happened today...

Some amazing things that happened today...

What could I have done to make today even better?

Date: ....

Quote Of The Day

Today I am truly grateful for...

Here's what would make today great...

I am...

Some amazing things that happened today...

Some amazing things that happened today...

What could I have done to make today even better?

Date: ....

Quote Of The Day

Today I am truly grateful for...

Here's what would make today great...

I am...

Some amazing things that happened today...

Some amazing things that happened today...

What could I have done to make today even better?

Date: ....

Quote Of The Day

____
____

Today I am truly grateful for...

____
____
____
____

Here's what would make today great...

____
____
____
____
____

I am...

____
____

Some amazing things that happened today...

____
____

Some amazing things that happened today...

____
____

What could I have done to make today even better?

____
____

Date: ....

Quote Of The Day

Today I am truly grateful for...

Here's what would make today great...

I am...

Some amazing things that happened today...

Some amazing things that happened today...

What could I have done to make today even better?

Date: ....

Quote Of The Day

Today I am truly grateful for...

Here's what would make today great...

I am...

Some amazing things that happened today...

Some amazing things that happened today...

What could I have done to make today even better?

Date:

Quote Of The Day

Today I am truly grateful for...

Here's what would make today great...

I am...

Some amazing things that happened today...

Some amazing things that happened today...

What could I have done to make today even better?

Date: ....

Quote Of The Day

Today I am truly grateful for...

Here's what would make today great...

I am...

Some amazing things that happened today...

Some amazing things that happened today...

What could I have done to make today even better?

Date: ____________

Quote Of The Day

Today I am truly grateful for...

Here's what would make today great...

I am...

Some amazing things that happened today...

Some amazing things that happened today...

What could I have done to make today even better?

Date: _______________

Quote Of The Day

Today I am truly grateful for...

Here's what would make today great...

I am...

Some amazing things that happened today...

Some amazing things that happened today...

What could I have done to make today even better?

Date: ____________

Quote Of The Day

Today I am truly grateful for...

Here's what would make today great...

I am...

Some amazing things that happened today...

Some amazing things that happened today...

What could I have done to make today even better?

Date: ....

Quote Of The Day

Today I am truly grateful for...

Here's what would make today great...

I am...

Some amazing things that happened today...

Some amazing things that happened today...

What could I have done to make today even better?

Date: _______________

Quote Of The Day
____
____
____

Today I am truly grateful for...
____
____
____
____
____

Here's what would make today great...
____
____
____
____
____

I am...
____
____
____

Some amazing things that happened today...
____
____

Some amazing things that happened today...
____
____
____

What could I have done to make today even better?
____
____

Date: ....

Quote Of The Day

Today I am truly grateful for...

Here's what would make today great...

I am...

Some amazing things that happened today...

Some amazing things that happened today...

What could I have done to make today even better?

Date:

Quote Of The Day

Today I am truly grateful for...

Here's what would make today great...

I am...

Some amazing things that happened today...

Some amazing things that happened today...

What could I have done to make today even better?

Date: ....

Quote Of The Day

Today I am truly grateful for...

Here's what would make today great...

I am...

Some amazing things that happened today...

Some amazing things that happened today...

What could I have done to make today even better?

Date: _______________

Quote Of The Day

____

____

____

Today I am truly grateful for...

____

____

____

____

____

Here's what would make today great...

____

____

____

____

____

I am...

____

____

____

Some amazing things that happened today...

____

____

Some amazing things that happened today...

____

____

What could I have done to make today even better?

____

____

Date:

Quote Of The Day

Today I am truly grateful for...

Here's what would make today great...

I am...

Some amazing things that happened today...

Some amazing things that happened today...

What could I have done to make today even better?

Date: ....

Quote Of The Day

Today I am truly grateful for...

Here's what would make today great...

I am...

Some amazing things that happened today...

Some amazing things that happened today...

What could I have done to make today even better?

Date: ______________________

Quote Of The Day

Today I am truly grateful for...

Here's what would make today great...

I am...

Some amazing things that happened today...

Some amazing things that happened today...

What could I have done to make today even better?

Date: ....

Quote Of The Day

Today I am truly grateful for...

Here's what would make today great...

I am...

Some amazing things that happened today...

Some amazing things that happened today...

What could I have done to make today even better?

Date: ....

Quote Of The Day

Today I am truly grateful for...

Here's what would make today great...

I am...

Some amazing things that happened today...

Some amazing things that happened today...

What could I have done to make today even better?

Date:

Quote Of The Day

Today I am truly grateful for...

Here's what would make today great...

I am...

Some amazing things that happened today...

Some amazing things that happened today...

What could I have done to make today even better?

Date: ....

Quote Of The Day

Today I am truly grateful for...

Here's what would make today great...

I am...

Some amazing things that happened today...

Some amazing things that happened today...

What could I have done to make today even better?

Date:

Quote Of The Day

Today I am truly grateful for...

Here's what would make today great...

I am...

Some amazing things that happened today...

Some amazing things that happened today...

What could I have done to make today even better?

Date: ....

Quote Of The Day

Today I am truly grateful for...

Here's what would make today great...

I am...

Some amazing things that happened today...

Some amazing things that happened today...

What could I have done to make today even better?

Date:

Quote Of The Day

Today I am truly grateful for...

Here's what would make today great...

I am...

Some amazing things that happened today...

Some amazing things that happened today...

What could I have done to make today even better?

Date: ....

Quote Of The Day

Today I am truly grateful for...

Here's what would make today great...

I am...

Some amazing things that happened today...

Some amazing things that happened today...

What could I have done to make today even better?